My
Horrible
C-Section

By: Lisa Bedrick

A Second Family

About two years ago I hit a deer with my car while on a pizza delivery. It messed up my car so much that it was barely working. The break pedal became almost impossible to push. I asked God why he let that happen to me. He said it was so I would be ready to start a family again. I wasn't ready then, so I sold that car and got a smaller, more fuel efficient car so I could keep doing pizza deliveries. I had to endure a bit more work drama and another demeaning boss before I was ready.

All women have to decide how they will contribute to society. Some do it with having children. Others do it with having a great career that they feel happy doing. I have done almost every job out there. I have seen the world, which I wanted to do before having kids. There is nothing else I wanted to accomplish. So I was ready for family number two to begin.

I resented a few times that I had to start at square one again. My ex refused to work things out with me. He refused to let me see my first two daughters. So I had to start over. I have realized lately though that he and I never really loved each other. He was not capable of love, for whatever reason. I therefore did not love him because I felt he did not love me.

I think as you get older you become more capable of love. When you are young, you don't know what love is. You think love is just passion, but it is generosity and humility. It is forgetting about yourself and putting the other person first. It is never wanting to hurt them in any way. It took me 35 years to figure out love. I suppose some never figure it out.

Family number 2 began in a very difficult way. I had a C Section 2 months ago. It was the hardest week of my life. It all started when my mother in law came over and noticed I looked off. She took my blood pressure and it was very high. She suggested that I go to the hospital. Luckily I was mentally prepared for this. I had been reading about presclampsia and realized that I might have that. My pee had foam in it for awhile, and I realized that probably was not normal. I read that babies can be and should be delivered early in such situations. But I was worried my baby would be in the ICU for awhile. Praise God he came out healthy. He was about 2 weeks early, but he was ok. At first they tried to induce my labor. That wasn't working, so 12 hours after they tried that I had a C section done. I guess before the C Section I said to the nurses, "Can we just get this over with?" So they did. It all seemed like a dream, but it was real. At that point I had been infused with God knows how many drugs. I was not myself. I kept trying to get off my hospital bed before the C Section, but my boyfriend wouldn't let me. He had a very firm look on his face as if to say, "No we are doing this." I'm sure my instincts kicked in and I was thinking, "Why am about to let them cut me open? That is crazy." So I was trying to escape.

But it happened. I had the C Section. The pain was quite annoying afterwards. I had a hard time getting up to pee and walking arond. I was walking like a turtle, which is funny because now I have 5 pet turtles. I wish I could say to them, "I was just like you a little bit ago." I survived though. That is all that matters. They put me on a ton of blood pressure medication that caused me to hallucinate a bit. They were all silly halluciations like worm people falling over each other. I don't recommend that anyone takes that. It really is just acid, I think anyways. Like acid off the street. It did not help my bloood pressure at all. What did help was getting home and sleeping more and eating good foods. God kept telling me to drink lots of juice, so I have been doing that for 2 months now. I just live off of juice, and yogurt and salads. That is how I got my blood pressure back to normal.

I never thought I would have a C Section. Ever since I started my period at 12 I have been horribly afraid of getting pregnant and having a C Section. But I did it. I overcame, and I am very proud of myself for surviving all that. If you ever need a C Section, I promise you too will be ok. Just believe that you will be ok and you will be.

Co-Sleeping

This is a very delicate topic when it comes to babies and kids. Should parents sleep in the same bed as their kids? If the child is older there is almost no risk of the child being injured. The key is that the parent needs to not be drunk or high or on any medication. Any parent that is under the influence of a drug should of course, never sleep in the same bed with a child or baby. If you are fully aware of your surroundings and your mind is working well, I think it's ok. It is ideal if one side of the bed is against a wall so the child cannot roll off. It can be safe and a great reward for being a parent if the cuddle time is done carefully.

To deprive a good parent who isn't on any substances of cuddling with their child is very sad. Most moms would never accidentally smother or injure their child. Their instincts from how much they love the child would prevent them from injuring the child.

My theory is that some moms can't handle being a mom. In their frustration over the baby crying, they hurt the baby. Then they say it was an accident. No I guarantee it was not an accident. They know themselves what their intentions were.

If you don't have the patience to raise a baby, then don't try doing it. It does take a lot of patience and self-sacrifice and loving others more than you love yourself. It is not a job that everyone should do. This is why some women get post-partum depression. They get overwhelmed with having to care for a little baby. It isn't easy. But it is fun and worth it.

The line I keep thinking of in regards to motherhood is from a Coldplay song, "Nobody said it was easy."

If you want to cuddle with your baby or your older child, do it. Just make sure you aren't drunk or high or on a substance. If your mind is clear, it is safe. That is my opinion.

May God bless all you fellow parents out there with patience and a great love for your baby or child. And may you never hurt your child because, obviously, you would regret doing that a lot.

The AC

When you have kids, of course you want to create the best possible environment for them. I have been wondering if running the AC hard is good or bad for my little baby.

 A few days ago my AC vent in my room was leaking. Not a lot, just a bit. We live in a slightly older home. It was probably built in the 60's. I thought about calling the AC repair guys, but then figured I could just not run the AC so hard. That seems to have fixed the leaking problem.

From now on I will set it at 74 during the day, maybe 76 if it's super hot outside. At night instead of 68 I'll put it at 71.

Lately it has been 106 every day here in Texas. Killer temps for sure. I felt like God said he was punishing the city I'm in. There are a lot of bad people here. Maybe the crazy high temps will make all the evil people go live somewhere else. I live in Odessa. For several years this city was the highest crime city in the entire U.S.

Why do I live here? I came here to try to see my daughters again. That didn't work out, but maybe someday it will. I could have lived in Florida, but with the humidity that may have felt just as hot.

I have always wondered if the AC puts out toxic chemicals. In one place I lived there was a sign on the AC unit that said it can cause cancer. So if you run your AC hard all day, I recommend you run it more lightly. The less toxic chemicals in the air, the better.

I think it is also wise to crack at least one window at night to let some fresh air in and let those chemicals out. You may have less allergy problems and less headaches. Fresh air is always nice to breath in.

I hope you all are enjoying your AC this summer and that it keeps working. But watch out for the side effects of it and try to run it not so strong. It is less drain on the power grid, and your lungs will thank you someday.

Watch Out for Conflict

 The cause of pretty much every conflict, and most parting of the ways of two people, is when two people want two totally different things.

For example, and this is a sad analogy, but my dad wanted to get physical with me as a kid, but I didn't obviously. So that created conflict and a parting of the ways for us.

My ex wanted me to have a 3rd kid, because he was dying to have a son. I didn't really want to. That was probably the main reason we parted ways. I figured the two lovely girls I already gave him should have been enough.

My ex mother in law really wanted to vaccinate my girls. I didn't want that, at all. So we stopped being friends because of that.

The only thing my best friend and I have conflicted over is I think she should try online dating, but she really doesn't want to. Otherwise we agree on pretty much anything. That is why we have stayed friends for 23 years.

My mom and I haven't conflicted on too much. I didn't really want her to marry my step dad but she did anyways. Once she was married, I didn't disagree with her over it anymore. It was already done.

Anytime two people want two very different things, there will be conflict. The way to avoid this is to pretty much never want anything, at least not a lot.

Watch out for wanting something that is totally different from what others want, within reason. If you know what is best, stick with that. Maybe you can change the mind of the other person to want what you want. If you can't, just let it go. Whatever you want so bad, just let it go. Then you will never have conflict ever again. Very nice.

A Crazy Guy named Eric

 The most crazy guy I have ever known was not my ex-husband. It was my ex bf. I can't believe I considered having kids with him a few times. I could tell he was crazy when I noticed he didn't wear socks. Who wears shoes without socks? That is disgusting.

The other odd thing was he was giving every dollar he made to his mom when I first met him. She was a millionaire supposedly. She didn't need the money. But he had a gambling problem, so he didn't trust himself to have more than $10 in his bank account at all times. If he had more, he would go play poker or gamble in some other way. After he was with me a while, he asked his mom for all his money back. I guess I helped him recover from that issue. His mom kept 4k of his money and gave him the other 40k back. He was shocked that she kept some. I was like, "Well that was her accounting fee I guess." He said she mentioned doing something like that once.

No matter how much he had, he always acted like he was broke. That may have been because he was Jewish. How he was did teach me something about money though. The more rich you act, the more broke you will be. The more poor you act, the more rich you will be.

He used to be addicted to cocaine. Some girl introduced him to it when he was about 20. He couldn't afford to live on his own, so he lived with his mom and then his dad and then his grandma. They all kept kicking him out because he was stealing money from them. They all spoiled him and let him live with them for free. He didn't have to pay any of them rent because each of them was a millionaire. Jewish people know how to get rich.

When he was with me, he stopped using cocaine, but he drank 3 Monster drinks every day. Then he got terrible headaches, and he didn't know why. Of course it was from the energy drinks. You can't put that much poison in your body and expect to feel ok still. I read that if you have 6 Monster drinks in a day, it will kill you. Be careful with energy drinks ya'll.

Due to the energy drinks, he was always on edge. He seemed non stop mad about something. He had it pretty easy with me, so there was almost nothing for him to be mad about. He lived with me for free. He got us groceries sometimes and that was great. He tried being generous with me a few times, like offering to buy me a new phone, but I always turned down his offers. I don't know why. I suppose because I don't like taking anything from anyone. "There is no such thing as a free lunch." The more you accept from someone, the more you feel like you owe them. He was not the kind of person I wanted to feel like I owed anything to. He had a problem with being able to forgive. His ex possibly cheated on him, and he was still bitter at her the entire year I knew him. I wanted to tell him every day, "Just get over it man." I doubt that would have helped though. He constantly watched videos about Narcissism to convince himself that she was the main one with the issues. He had issues too, but narcissists never look in the mirror. They see what is wrong with everyone else but never themselves. That is why people like him never get any better.

The craziest thing he ever did was threaten to drop me off on the side of the road on our way back from 6 Flags. I don't think I did anything that bad. I was just being quiet. That seems to really annoy people if you won't talk to them in the car. I remember another ex going psycho on me for being silent in the car. Why do you always have to talk in the car? I don't think anyone should have to if they don't feel like talking. Most likely it was just that the driving was bothering them. I really like driving. Some people hate driving. Those people should just stay home I would say.

I have had lots of drama with all my exes. I finally found a peace loving man and a calm place to call home. Thank God my man knows how to stay in peace. I hope we will always maintain a peaceful and happy home.

May God bless you all with a peaceful home. Keep it peaceful.

Jealousy Over Children

 I think it is very common that husbands are jealous of the love between a mother and a son. Women also get jealous of the love between a father and a daughter.

Perhaps each parent wonders if that kid will replace them emotionally someday. That happens quite often. A woman might love her son more than her man. A father may begin to love his daughter more than his wife.

Obviously that is not good if that happens. I heard in sermons a lot, "A marriage is forever. Kids are only for 18 years. You need to love your spouse more than you love your kids." Also if you forget about loving your spouse and focus on the kids, that marriage won't last very long.

It is always a balancing act for every mom. She needs to try showing equal love to her man and her kids. It can be quite tricky to do that.

I named my son James. I realized after that the meaning of that name is "supplanter" or replacer. To me that means it could be easy for me to let my baby boy replace my man in my heart. I need to watch out for that.

Spouses are supposed to be the first priority, then children.

The love a parent has for their child needs to be in light of knowing they won't be around forever. Someday they will fall in love and run away from you, emotionally. That transition will be a lot smoother if you don't let them into your heart too much in the first place. Then you will be more ok with them falling in love and leaving you. ☹

When it is time to, let your kids go. Realize that your call to parent is only temporary. Always and forever keep your mate as your first priority. They deserve that.

Mom Attachment

 This may seem odd, but every time my bf talks to his mom in person or texts her I feel jealous. Why do I feel that way? I now know why. Because my ex husband basically left me to go marry his mom. I have always heard the Oedipus complex says that every man wants to kill his father and marry his mother. Ewe...

Emotionally Ben was married to his mom his whole life. I never mattered as much as she did. He wanted me to look like his mom and raise my kids like she would. Ultimately I think he felt she should take over mothering my kids because he knew he liked her more.

So I have mother in law issues. I really like my current mother in law though. She is a great person. But we all have our own baggage to deal with. The first cut is the deepest.

When I met my ex-husband Ben, the doors on his closet were all over his room. I asked, "What happened to your closet doors?" He said, "Oh my mom said it looks better that way." To me that proved she was crazy.

We lived with her for a few months before our first baby was born. She would pace the hallway at 2am and move things around. It may have been due to a medication she was on. I did not get why she wouldn't just go to sleep.

One time we were going on a road trip to CA so Ben could meet my parents. His mom texted and called him non stop to try to stop us from going. Maybe she feared that we would stay there forever. I wish we would have. Maybe our marriage would have lasted longer.

She babysat our two girls for one week so we could have a beach vacation. At the end of the week she texted me a text meant for her daughter. It said, "She didn't even ask how the girls were all week." I think she was gossiping trying to say I didn't care about my daughters at all. Gossip was her favorite hobby.

And here I am basically gossiping about her. The moral to this story is, don't be an annoying mother in law. Respect it that your child needs to move on. You should not run their life anymore. They need to bond with their mate and let go of you, so let them. Cut off those apron strings and let your kids be adults.

Doctors

I saw a great quote on Facebook a while ago. It said, "Doctors are the same are robbers. They both cut you open and take all your money." :)

A ton of people worship doctors. As in they pretty much put doctors in the place of God. :(Why? The reason is because at some point either they or their child was in serious need of having their life saved, and a doctor saved their life. From then on, without realizing it, they decided to worship doctors.

Doctors have saved my life a few times. Once I fell off my bike on my face when I was about 6. It was a very hard fall. My face was covered in blood. If doctors did not stitch my gums up, I most likely would have bled to death.

Another time when I was 12 my appendix got infected and it exploded. Doctors saved my life and cleaned up my insides from all the appendix poison. On a side note though, I have wondered lately if that happened after my multiple Hep B vaccines right before that. I remember thinking even as a kid, "Why do I need this shot multiple times? That seems shady."

Then a few years ago I had gall stones. Doctors again saved my life by taking out my gall bladder. If they hadn't done that, I probably would have died.

After all that, do I choose to worship doctors? No. I am grateful for them. But I will never worship them. I only worship God. God saved me through those doctors. It wasn't just the doctors that saved me. God does miracles today through healthcare.

The problem though is that God allows Satan also to work through healthcare. I had an ex a while ago who told me, "Doctors don't want you to get well. They want you to stay sick so they can make more money off of you." He ironically died due to doctors. He was prescribed one too many pills and it was just too much for his body to handle. He was on an anti-depressant called Klonopin, Cialis to fix the side effects of the Klonopin, Testosterone shots, and the day he died, a random clinic doctor gave him anti-biotics. He was just sneezing a lot that day. That was his only symptom. :(That night he went out drinking and he died. It wasn't just the drinking that killed him. It was drinking and having way too many pills in his body. None of the doctors made it super clear that drinking in addition to all those pills could be deadly. Maybe back then, 10 years ago, they just didn't know. Some people don't care. They take pills and drink as if they want to die. In that case, it isn't just the doctors who are to blame, obviously.

Overall, are doctors to be worshipped? No of course not. They are not God. They may act like they are. They may want you to believe everything they say without questioning it. But you can be smart too. Maybe you didn't go to 12 years of college, but you can be just as wise as them if you want to be. Just do the research on what you need to research so you can be wise too.

Don't ever worship doctors. Only worship God.

Heartburn

 The hardest part about pregnancy is heartburn. It isn't the difficulty with getting out of bed or the crazy pain in your back. It is the terrible heartburn that you get when you are tired at night. I still get it sometimes when I am tired. I never know if eating or not eating is the best thing to do when I have it.

I never struggled with heartburn until my last pregnancy. I remember my ex was always taking Zantac for his heartburn. I figured he ate too much fried chicken and burgers, and he probably did. That definitely can make it worse. The best cure, I noticed, is drinking milk and having a whole wheat muffin when the heartburn hits. It also helps a lot to use a heating pad on your chest. Not the kind you warm up, but the electrical kind that stays really hot. Heat is good for all kinds of health issues.

I watched a video called, "Cancer Can be Cured." The cancer patients went to Germany and got high infusions of vitamin C and heat treatments. Those two things cured their cancer. Also eating a lot more vegetables. Then they didn't need chemo and their cancer went away. Pretty great.

For heartburn, I also tried putting icy hot patches on my chest right where it hurt. That seemed to permanently fix it. The kind I buy are Salonpas. They are cheap and are made in Japan. For any pain I have, I put one of those on it and the pain goes away. My neck was killing me the other day and one of those fixed it. Try getting those.

The best way to prevent heartburn is to eat healthy. Eat a salad every day. Drink a smoothie every day. Try to eat only foods that you know your body will love. Then you will be much less likely to get heartburn. Also an apple a day keeps the doctor away, and heartburn.

How to Loose Weight After a Baby Delivery

 Here is a sad story. My aunt got a tummy tuck after having her first son. The really sad part about that is that her husband was and is 300 pounds. Why should he care if she looked slightly overweight after having a baby, when he was that big? I hate when men expect their woman to look perfect always when they don't. That is not fair. The reverse is true too I suppose. If a woman doesn't try to stay thin, she should not expect her man to stay thin either.

It is hard for anyone to lose weight. The hard thing about losing weight after having a baby is that you have to take care of the baby in the middle of the night. In order to do so in a happy mood, you need to eat to have more energy. Maybe that is why post partum women don't lose weight that fast. It could be stress eating. It is also just eating to have the energy to work harder.

It helps to go on walks to lose weight. Getting a part time job as a waitress or a store stocker can help too. I might work in retail soon being a stocker. I'm sure that will help for me to get my baby weight off. It does bother me sometimes.

I think that's why the women who don't have kids, don't. They don't want to worry about all the extra weight from pregnancy and wanting to get rid of it. I think it is also why some women just have one baby after another. They probably think, "Well I'm fat already so why not get pregnant again and get more fat?" But you can get that weight off. It is possible. Just try harder.

Obviously, it is ideal to avoid candy, cookies and chips. If you do eat chips, I recommend pringles. I am currently re-kindling my love of pringles. At least they don't hurt my stomach after eating them, so they can't be that bad for you.

If you crave chocolate, try chocolate covered almonds. I read that almonds are the number one super food, meaning they prevent cancer and any other disease you probably never want to get.

Drink lots of water. Often times when we think we are hungry, we are actually just thirsty. Drink juice a lot. The main thing God told me to use to cure my high blood pressure was orange juice. Orange juice is ideal, but any juice helps with any illness you have. The vitamin C is very much needed for your organs.

Be patient with yourself getting that baby weight off. All good things take effort. You will be movie star attractive again eventually. Just be patient.

Hug Your Baby

 A lot of people know that babies need to be hugged to burp them, but it's good to hug them at other times too. Babies need a lot of interaction and affection. I try to always keep my baby where he can see me. I try to never leave him alone for very long.

I remember hearing about something called Ferberizing your baby, meaning let them cry and learn to self sooth. That is just ridiculous. All babies need parents. That is why we are here. Babies cannot self sooth. Either they need a bottle or a diaper or to be rocked to sleep. They don't know how to make themselves happy yet. They are totally dependent on adults. No one can expect a baby to just help itself.

Make sure that you stay attentive to your baby. They almost always need something. It is like working 2 full time jobs to do a good job caring for a baby. If they don't need a bottle, they need a diaper. If it's not that, they need to burp. If it's none of those, they need to be rocked to sleep. They generally cannot fall asleep on their own. It would be great if they could, but they can't.

The better job you do in meeting a baby's needs, the more they will learn to trust the world. If a baby is not helped every time they need help, they will grow up angry or sad.

Make sure to give your baby lots of hugs. It is just as good for you as it is for them. If you have to change your clothes 6 times a day from them spitting up on your shoulder, oh well. It helps you learn to enjoy doing laundry.

Our CPS Fiasco

I think it's possible my ex called CPS on me to mess up my current family. I don't know for sure. It may have been a seperate thing. But something tells me it was related to him and his evil mother. I hope my two daughters will not turn out to be anything like that woman.

My ex had always wanted a son. I just had a son finally, with my new mate. I posted pics on Twitter when I was still in the hospital about him being born. The next morning, a lady from CPS visited my room to talk about "accusations." She did ask me if I had other kids and why I didn't have them in my custody. Later we had a family meeting with them with my current family. They asked me a lot of questions about my daughters. I simply said my ex was difficult, and that is why I don't see my daughters.

I suppose it seems odd to any woman for a mom to not see her kids. Usually the absent mom is on drugs in such cases. I have never done serious drugs. I used to think working at Papa John's was my drug, and workaholism can be a drug. I simply have not seen them for a long time, because I don't want to see my ex or his mom. I don't care for either of them anymore. I don't care to see them.

I am a bit grateful to them for caring for my girls, but mostly I hate it that they stole them from me and have never said sorry. My ex mother in law stopped talking to my mom about a year ago for no reason. So now we are all in the dark as to how they are doing, and they don't seem to care at all. They are the most heartless and godless family I have ever known. I hate that they are raising my daughters now, but I have no control over that. Someday I may get a lawyer and try to get my girls back but not now. I hope my daughters are doing ok and are healthy. And I hope my ex and his mother fully realize how Lucky they are to get to care for them. They better never take caring for my girls for granted.

Getting a Son

All men want a son. For some sad reason, men never seem to want a girl. Maybe they feel girls have less value. A son might go to work someday and bring the family more money. Girls can do that too though, just want to point that out. Girls can make just as much as men if they are determined to do so.

Why does God allow only some men to have a son? The more capable a man is of being a great leader, the more likely that God will give him a son. To have a son is a big compliment from God. It is God's reward to good men who are honest and kind and have great morals. God does not want boys to imitate bad men. Therefore only good men get to have sons.

It is odd to me that my dad got to have a son. I don't get why. I know he had tons of potential at first to be a strong leader and a godly role model. But then Satan invaded his mind and he fell down hard due to sexual sins. Great men often fall, because the world hates strong men. Why do they? Because they are jealous of strong men.

Only the lucky few men are blessed with having a son. If you want a son, always be the kind of man that God wants to bless with a boy. Always maintain a strong, hard work ethic so you can show your son how to work hard. Honor and submit to God so that you can teach your son how to submit to God. Be the kind of man that our future generation should want to imitate.

In Laws

It is tricky to have in laws. Everyone, almost, has a hard time with their in laws. It is just awkward because you have to pretend they are your family when they really aren't. Luckily with my in laws, my mother in law looks like my aunt and my grandmother in law looks like my late grandma. So that is nice. I feel like I have known them my entire life.

My ex in laws did not remind me of anyone. They were people that I never saw eye to eye with and I never could understand them. They never took my ex to church as a kid. I had ongoing resentment at them for that. No wonder he went crazy from his demons. He did not have a good foundation at all. Take your kids to church. Their future mate will very much thank you for doing that.

My current man was put in private Christian school from a young age. He was taken to church a lot. That was the main reason I picked him, actually. Most parents do not care that much about their kids to put them in private school. I knew when I heard about that that I would like them overall.

I feel I have a good relationship with my in laws. Hopefully it will always stay good.

Expectations

I realized recently that my mom never said to me, "When are you going to give me grandkids?" You always see that in movies. I think it was after my dad sexually molested me that she gave up any dream of a perfect family being possible. Her parents were mostly happy. They stayed married for 65 years, but they fought a lot. My grandpa was abusive to the kids. Maybe my mom had wanted a very different life for me. She wasn't waiting to marry me off like all the moms in Jane Austen novels. She wanted me to go to college and finish maybe so I could run my own life. I think she wanted me to never be dependent on a man. But I still have been, and it has been a fun ride.

In high school and college my grandma would always ask me, "Do you have a boyfriend." I would say, "No." She would say, "Good, keep it that way." I think she wanted me to avoid marriage if I could.

I realized a while ago that I have never seen a truly happy marriage. My grandparents seemed happy on the outside, but I knew they were not. My mom and dad seemed happy, but if they were, why did he molest me? My mom and step-dad never seemed happy. I always saw them as just roommates living together. There was not much love between them.

A lot of couples resign to that though, just being roommates. The passion fades. The enamor you may have felt goes away after they say or do a few dumb things. The love cools off. You stay friends, but there is less excitement the longer you are with them. You no longer stare at them while they sleep. You aren't dying for them to come home like you used to. But who can sustain that kind of infatuation for long? It can feel like idolatry, which I think is why it fades for most couples. They feel maybe that is wrong to be that obsessed with another person.

We all have expectations for love and marriage and raising children, but eventually we change our expectations to be more realistic. The reason people get mad about anything is because they are not willing to change their expectations. What do you deserve? What do they deserve? It is nice to do the best you can, but that is all you can do. That is all they can do.

Motherhood is often something girls dream about. We grow up thinking, "I'll be the perfect mom someday." But there is no perfect mom. It is not possible to be perfect. We do the best we can. I felt very disappointed in myself for not giving my current child more breast milk. I tried nursing a few times. I think he was just too weak because he was a primi. I tried pumping a lot. It was a very slow process. Usually I felt I needed sleep more then I needed to pump myself. But then I felt guilty for not giving him more breast milk. I felt God tell me a few times to let myself off the hook for that.

It is so hard to care for your man and your child and yourself, but it's important to figure out how to do that. Women often only think of the needs of others, and we tend to neglect ourselves. That is one reason I allow myself to buy a few fun things every week that will make me happy. I think all mothers needs to do that, so they can still get things they want too. Food doesn't really make me happy, but solar powered lights do. :) If you give and give and give, eventually you will burn out. It is good to reward yourself in some way for all that you do.

Don't worry too much if you don't do everything you were hoping to do as a mother. It takes time to become a great mom. We all struggle in various ways. We need help. Accept the help that others try to give you. Give yourself breaks to relax. Try to still get outside. Get a stroller to take your baby outside. Remember that you are doing the best you can and be kind to yourself. Positive self talk will make your days go a lot better.

Death

Back in the day a ton of women would die in child labor or after giving birth. I am very lucky that my baby and I survived. My blood pressure was the highest they had seen at the hospital. A doctor came to talk with me after the C Section. He said how my blood pressure was so high I could have died from a stroke or a heart attack. I just shrugged like what was I supposed to do about it. I ate mostly healthy in my pregnancy. Toward the end I had Sprite for a few weeks. I may have eaten too many hot dogs. Maybe those two things seriously messed up my body. My arms were hurting a lot. I think I developed arthritis in my arms from my hard work at Papa John's. They seemed to have a flare up when I was pregnant. A flare up is a good term because they felt on fire. I also possibly wrote too many books last winter and that worsened my arthritis. It is a miracle that I didn't die in my last pregnancy from high blood pressure. In the hospital they asked me, "Are you in pain or are you tired?" I said, "I'm always in pain, and I'm always tired." I think almost my entire life I have always had pain somewhere in my body, and I have always been tired. I think everyone is tired all the time or else why do people live on soda or coffee? It seems that my neck or my back or my feet always hurt. That is because I always work hard cleaning or doing some fun project. Such is life.

One thing that may have caused my blood pressure to go up is that I literally prayed to die while I was pregnant. That was the first time in my life that I prayed that. I am sure a lot of women have done that. You get tired of peeing 10 times every night and the extremely painful heartburn. It is very hard to get out of bed toward the end. It was winter most of my pregnancy, so the grass was brown, and the house was cold and that made me sad. I missed my two daughters a lot. I am so grateful now that they are mostly replaced by my son, but it was hard to not have my daughters the past 4 years. That is not normal, and it was very difficult. I wanted to die, but now I feel a lot better. Now that my son is here I have a reason to want to stay alive. He is so wonderful.

Hopefully my life will be happy from here on out. Hopefully I will be glad to be alive every day, and I will be more grateful for all that I have, rather then focused on what I lost. May God help me to stay strong and healthy the rest of my life.

 I had to deal with a bunny dying a few days ago. I was quite shaken up over it. It was the third time I have had a bunny die. Each time I figured it was my cat or another cat that scared it and gave it a heart attack. Poor little bunny. Or they could not find the water. Or they didn't realize how much water they needed to drink in the Texas heat. I let my bunnies run free in my backyard. I think it's mean to shut them up in a cage. But then they have to make sure and drink lots of water. The more they run around, the more water they need.

Anyways, I still have 5. I had gotten 6. My plan is to breed them and sell the babies for $50 each. It couldn't hurt to have some more cash coming in. I just hope the babies will make it. I have a cat and 3 kittens also. The mom bunny will need to hide the babies really well so the cats won't find them. Maybe she won't eat them and she will realize they are pets. I give her wet cat food twice a day so that might prevent her from eating any adult or baby bunnies. I could give her away, but there are neighbor cats who come in our backyard too. One of them is so funny. He looks super scared every time he is back there, like he thinks I might shoot him for coming onto my property. I think he is friends with my girl cat. He seems to be a step dad to the kittens too. Their dad was a black cat. I think its owners moved away recently so he is gone too. Another black dad abandoning his kids.

The only other animal I had die was my rat named Ratty when I was little. I buried him in our front yard. That was sad. There is nothing more creepy then realizing an animal is stiff and dead. I have never seen a dead person, praise God for that. I had an ex die but it wasn't at our apartment. He died at his friend's house on his couch from drinking too much. I can only imagine how traumatizing that must have been for his friend to discover his stiff body in the morning. He shouldn't have pressured him to go to the bar the night before. I had helped my ex quit drinking for a year. Then that stupid "friend" convinced him to go to a bar one night and he died. Bars are evil. Don't go to them.

I have not talked to my two daughters in over 3 years. Partly because I wanted to move on from my past and because my ex is difficult. One friend said that seems suspicious though, like my ex is trying to hide something. I keep wondering if they are both dead now. I know my ex's family was all about vaccines. They took my oldest to get 5 shots in one day, almost like they wanted her to die. If you don't care about a kid, by all mean give them as many shots and meds as you want. If you want them to stay alive, keep their body clean of any man-made substances.

Life is so fragile. When my ex died I realized that could happen to me at any time. He was only 34 when he died. I realized that I wanted to accomplish a lot before I died and got started doing it. I started this blog, and then published tons of books. By now it has been about 30 books. Not to brag but I am glad I finished that goal. I just wanted to publish at least one book before I died.

My only other goal before I die is to do a cruise around South America. That may be possible soon. I think that would be the most fun thing I will have ever done in my life. Can't wait! I also have an ongoing dream of living in Northern CA. I got to do a class at Berkeley one summer. We went hiking all over that area, and it was so pretty. I hope to live around there someday with my new little family. I actually had a great dream last night that I was moving back to CA.

Whatever you want to do before you die, get it done. Don't put it off for too long. You never know how much more time you could have left.

Child Spanking

 For some reason, the majority of American parents now think that spanking is child abuse, but there is the verse, "Spare the rod, spoil the child." We wonder why so many kids now don't respect adults. It's because they were not spanked. If you want your kid to respect you, you have to spank them. Not a ton. Please don't spank them over just little things. Pick your battles. Meaning only spank when they do something seriously wrong. For example, my daughter was spanked for taking her seatbelt off and pushing her little sister down. There can be a fine line between good discipline and child abuse. Some parents discipline too much. Other parents like to never spank at all, which can be just as bad for the child.

It takes energy and courage to discipline your child. You might say you don't want to abuse them, but really you don't have the courage to discipline them. You have to show any kid who the boss is, you. They are not the boss of you. You are the boss of them. Today kids are in charge of the home instead of the parents. It is very sad. I don't know how that happened, but that is why most kids are spoiled now. Most

American children now are totally spoiled, selfish and narcissistic. You have to spank that ego out of them.

Kids will most respect adults that force them to respect them. Kids do not naturally respect adults. You have to train them to respect you.

I spanked my oldest daughter. She needed more spankings than my younger daughter. I feel a bit bad now because she possibly had slight autism. It is possible she couldn't help what she was doing. But you could say that about any kid. They don't know any better, so you have to train them.

I think with most autistic kids, the parents feel they can't discipline them. They make excuses for the kid. Just because their brain is defective, that doesn't mean you can't treat them like other children. All children need to be disciplined. I think autistic children only get worse when they are just allowed to do whatever they want to do. I'm not saying it's easy to control such children, but the parents still need to try. If there is no control over children, our society will lead to anarchy, essentially.

Make sure your kids respect you. It helps if you respect yourself. The more you respect yourself, the more you will know your kids need to respect you, and the more you will desire that they respect you.

Porn Kills Families

In most cases of divorce, the man leaves his wife and kids to go off and start a new family. I was watching Hope Floats again the other day. That is what happens in that movie. It usually is because the mom became too common. She stopped making herself look pretty. No matter how much a man loves a woman, he still wants her to look nice for him. The reverse is true too. Men, keep yourself looking hot for your wife. You can do it. :) Maybe the kids stress out the mom so she turns mean and grumpy. I used to always call my ex grumpy bear. He was more the one who got seriously grumpy after kids entered his life. I think he always hated how much he had to work, but that is what men with kids are meant to do. If you don't want to work hard, don't have kids.

I suppose family break ups also happen when both parents didn't totally want the kids. With my ex, he didn't really want kids. He said he did, just to get me probably, but he didn't seem to really want them. That was always an issue for us. I felt like a single mom the whole time I was married to him. He was just working and sleeping. I had to force him to interact with our girls. He was distraught over them being girls and not boys. What was the icing on the cake was when he told me he was watching porn. It then dawned on me, he was probably neglecting us for hours and just watching porn in his room. How can you keep a marriage going after knowing that? Some can make it through things like that but it's rare. My current bf kind of neglects me and our son, but it's to take care of his grandma. That is a much more noble reason.

Don't watch porn. It will mess up your marriage. If you want to watch porn, don't desire to be married. That is disrespectful to whoever you are with. It is saying to them that you would rather look at those bodies all day instead of your mate's body. And maybe you would, but that doesn't mean you should. The more you watch porn, the less satisfied you will be with your mate or with the sex life you two have.

I still have anger at my ex for doing that and keeping it secret for 7 years. I thought he was some great Christian guy. Just know ladies, no matter how good your man thinks he is or says he is, he might not be. Don't be an idiot and blindly trust him. I feel like an idiot for trusting my ex for 7 years.

When families break up, the adult leaving the kids isn't leaving the kids, he or she is leaving the mate. If the kids have to be ignored in order to ignore the ex, then that has to be done. I don't know how some divorced couples still talk "for the kids." If you don't like them enough to be married to them, don't talk to them. That's just weird. No one should talk to exes. It makes no sense.

Let the past go and let yourself be happy in your current life. Hopefully your past won't mess up your present.

Family Challenges

 When my brother was 19 he got his gf pregnant. They broke up. He didn't know he had a son until after his son was born. He tried shared custody but his ex was difficult. He then moved back to CA to be with my mom and I. From age 2 to 7 he didn't see his son. Then my grandpa told him to go back to NE and be a father to his son. I cried a ton when he left CA, but I was proud of him for forcing his ex to let him be a father to his son.

Now I am about to go 5 years without seeing my kids. I realized recently God gives us all 2 parents so we will always have at least 1. I lost my dad at age 14. I felt like 14 to 18, when I just had my mom, was the best time of my life. I can only hope my daughters are having the best time of their lives. It can be a lot better to just have 1 parent rather than 2.

Kids do tend to break couples up. I remember when my oldest was little, she would push my ex and I apart when we would hug. So we just stopped hugging. And that was the beginning of our great divide.

If you are a grandma, it helps a lot to watch the kids so the parents can have couple time. Kids are great, but they tend to divide their parents. I am surprised that any families stay together. May God help all the families to not get torn apart. And keep hugging your mate, even if your kids seem to not like it.

To my Ex's Family

Here is a blog I wrote that I hoped my ex and his family would read:

I have no idea if you all will read this, but I hope you know how evil you all are. You want me to pay child support, but you won't even let me see my kids? That makes no sense. If you want child support from me, you would have to allow me to see them every week. Why would I give you child support when you don't need it? If you all are working like you should be. "If a man will not work, he shall not eat."

I have always despised your extreme greed. "The love of money is the root of all evil" and you all love money far too much. Someday God will be done blessing you due to your extreme greed and pride. Seek first the kingdom of God and all those other things will be added to you.

I'm sorry I married Ben. He had many evil spirits due to Charismania that I finally saw. Being with him was the stupidest decision of my life. He was not good for me at all. That is why things never went well for us. But now you all get to be blessed with 2 wonderful girls. You're welcome. I have moved on and have a new life, since you wouldn't let me stay involved in their lives.

I hope you all stay healthy and I wish you well. Just pretend I don't exist like I have had to pretend you all don't exist. And take those girls to church. That is my final request in regards to them. Hopefully you all will find God someday too.

Nurses

After a woman has a baby, either naturally or a C Section, a nurse comes in her room and pushes hard on her abdomen like 10 times. They don't explain why the heck they are doing it. I swear they leave the room smiling after torturing you. It is supposedly to force the uterus to go back to normal. Why not let it contract naturally when it wants to?

This is why women still look pregnant after having a baby. The uterus is still pushed out. It's like the nurses could say, "We have to push that stomach back tight so your man will stay with you." I should have said, "Well that is plastic surgery that I did not ask for." Mainly with the nurses who did that to me I wanted to say, "Good Lord! Do you want my stitches to rip open?" They need to be more gentle. And smarter. Ah nurses....

They also drew my blood every day in the hospital. I asked, "Why do you need to keep drawing my blood?" They said, "We have to figure out why your blood pressure isn't going down after giving you all this medication." I wanted to say, "Because it doesn't work."

Of course my blood pressure probably also stayed high because they kept drawing my blood and pushing hard on my stomach.

 Hospitals are not easy. Every 20 minutes someone is in your room to talk to you about something. I told the nurses one time, "Maybe if you guys would let me take a nap, my blood pressure would get better."

In my second delivery I had a snotty nurse. She told me I wasn't actually in labor, even though I knew for a fact I was. She said I could either go back home or let them inject Pictocin into me. That speeds up the labor. I chose the Pictocin and my baby Joy came out one hour later. But she was blue and the umbilical cord was wrapped around her neck. Did that affect her later in life? I always saw her as very smart. She was talking well even before her older sister, for the most part. I don't think that fiasco made her less smart, but still I was always kind of mad that it happened. All because some snotty nurse could not be patient with my labor process.

One time a nurse was drawing my blood and handed me a vial of my blood while she tried to get more out. That freaked me out. I had asked them to run tests because I kept throwing up. It turned out it was just from stress. I was in college then. It may have also been my gall bladder dying, but they couldn't see that from just blood tests.

Another time I got my blood drawn, because my mom made me, which I resented. I was about 16. My arm got severely bruised due to the nurse fishing around for my veins. Just thinking of it now gives me chills.

Nurses, be nicer. I am sure your job is hard, but put yourself in the mindset and feelings of your patient. "Do to others as you would have them do to you."

And for all my fellow tortured victims, hang in there. This too shall pass. The nurses will let you be at peace eventually. Just eat healthy so they can't hurt you anymore.

Kids and Money

I used to tell my ex that when my girls grew up and got married we could live with them. I said that could be our retirement. He said that was stupid. I was thinking after all the waking up in the middle of the night for them, that didn't seem stupid to me.

All kids do owe their parents. They kept you alive for 18 years and provided all your needs. That is why God said, "Honor your mother and father."

I used to struggle with that given my dad and step-dad were child predators. It is never totally easy to honor your parents, but it's good in the long run if you can.

If your parent needs anything, you should help them, if you are able to do so.

The issue in our modern world is most parents are so rich, their kids know they won't have to help them. I suppose that is both a blessing and sad. Then families stay far apart when no one needs anyone else.

This is why poor families are somewhat cute. They all help each other a lot, because they all need help at some point. My grandma had to help my mom a lot when she was a single mom. I'm sure she appreciated her daughter asking for help. But now we all are so independent. Most people don't need other people for anything. This causes an isolation that causes the depression issue in our society. Very sad.

Vaccines

I debated with my ex and his mom for about a year about vaccines. I would get him on my side and then she would drag him back over to her side. Finally I lost the war and I let my ex's mom have my girls. I gave them up, because I got worn out trying to protect them from vaccines. My ex mother in law vaccinated my girls against my will, and I wish I knew how it affected their mental health. I have not seen them since they were vaccinated, and in a small way, I am scared to. I wonder if the vaccines gave them both Autism. In my generation most of the boys ended up with ADD, and I have always suspected if that was from the vaccines. Now because more shots are required for children, a lot of children become autistic. Most people just don't hear about it, because those families are paid to keep quiet.

After my first family debated about vaccines, it seemed like the entire world debated about vaccines. I was scared America would end up in a literal civil war over the Covid vaccine. Thank God we didn't. Thank God we all still like each other whether we got vaccinated or chose not to.

The main issue with vaccines is that you don't know who will have an "allergic reaction" to them until they do. You do not realize they are bad until it is too late. Although many parents, and people, heard that still small voice in their head telling them not to get a vaccine, to not allow a doctor to inject their child, they ignore the voice, and then they or their child has to face major health issues as a result.

Now I am in another debate with a new in law about vaccines. If only she would do the research, she would see they are evil. But she is a lemming just like most people are. She believes they are beneficial simply because she has heard they are. No second guessing. No praying about it. All she knows is that she thinks doctors are to be worshipped and normal people know pretty much nothing. That is her crazy belief system.

Ah...may God help all the overly compliant people in the world. Those who refuse to think for themselves. Make up your own mind people. What do you know to be true in your spirit? What is God saying to you about vaccines? Follow that. Not what you believe you should do. Only do what you know God tells you to do.

My Green Grass Project

Ever since I moved into my home over a year ago, I have had the goal to get grass all over the front and backyard. It literally is taking me more than a year. I live in a desert so it's hard to get anything to grow here. Most yards in this city are just dirt or half dirt.

I remember before I moved in here, I was in an apartment across the street. I used to look over at this street all the time. There was one house with super green grass. I always wondered how they kept their grass that green. Literally the grass was greener on the other side. It made me start dreaming about living in one of these houses. I had thought of renting one but figured I couldn't afford that on my own. Then I met my sweetie. In our first conversation he said, "I have a house over by where you live." I was thinking, "How can he have a house? He is only 30." He is part of a blessed family that I get to be a part of now too. The least I could do is help them get more grass.

Hopefully soon I'll get wonderful green grass everywhere here. It will be very exciting if it happens.

Substitutions

Here is my observation on my current family, Zach is the new Ben, Grandma Mary is the new Serenity, Margie is the new Joy and James is the new grandma Wanda. They are both an Aries sign.

I kept thinking of Ben's name when I thought of Zach because I finally love someone as much as I loved Ben. It took 4 years to find a sufficient replacement, but God helped me find Zach finally. Praise God.

Mary is Zach's grandma. She is just as strong in personality as Serenity was. Both were natural born leaders, fearless, confident, and have a strong desire to be helpful.

Margie is Zach's mom. She has a calm and friendly personality just like my youngest girl Joy. Both are super sweet and loving. I miss Joy. But at least now I have Margie to somewhat replace her.

James, my son, reminds me a lot of my grandma. It is like her spirit is in him. He always knows what he wants, like she did. You can tell he is very smart. From day 1 he was listening to me closely. I know someday he will be the leader of his family like my grandma always was for us.

People exit your life for many reasons, but God will replace them eventually.

Precious Memories

My mother in law is bringing a bouncer toy over for my baby boy today. I'm very excited about it. It reminds me of when I had Joy, my second girl. I would put her in her bouncer every morning and say, "Hi Joy," several times to her while I was making breakfast and washing their bottles. It was so cute. She would just smile and smile, like my baby boy smiles at me now in the mornings.

I think the smell of me making coffee makes him want to smile more. That makes sense.

Other good memories I have... I remember Joy poking our bunny in the eye multiple times. That was funny. He had black around his eye. Maybe she was just enthralled by how his eye looked. I remember Serenity going in circles around the driveway on her scooter and making it look like a circus act. The only thing we watched with a circus was Madagascar 3. It was adorable to see her do that. I remember her speeding down the street on her scooter, just as fast as a car would go. I was always amazed with her great athletic ability. If there was a scooter Olympics for kids, she would have won the gold medal for sure.

I remember doing exercise videos with Joy called Just Walk, or something like that. We would do the step aerobics together in the living room. It was adorable to see her do it with me. I remember taking the girls to the pool and them climbing up the ladder and jumping in the water into my arms. That was so cute.

When Serenity was a newborn, I took about 10 pictures of her every day in all kinds of outfits. She was my first child, so I was on cloud 9 having her. She made me so, so happy! Often times the flash was on with my phone so she would wince at the bright light flashing in her face. That was funny. I didn't know back then how to turn the flash off.

After Joy was born I went to pick her up at the hospital and I felt so much love for her. I have never felt so much love for anyone in my life. It might be because her birth was high risk. She came out blue with the umbilical cord around her neck. I think it was from the Pitocin they gave me to speed up my labor. I was so thankful that she made it and I promised her and myself I would take excellent care of her.

I felt a similar great compassion for my current baby. He was a primi and was only 5.5 pounds at birth. He was so skinny, but that made him so much cuter. I kept thinking he reminded me of my big brother who was always super skinny. I felt much closer to him for that reason. I promised him I would help him get fat quickly, and I did. He looks like a little football player now.

I remember I baptized Serentiy in a lake. I dunked her without fully explaining the whole thing. I think she thought I was trying to drown her. That was pretty funny. I mean I felt bad too, obviously. With Joy, I baptized her by just putting water on her head. I figured I should make it a more fun experience for her.

I remember going on bike rides with Serenity in a bike seat in front of me. With her helmet on she looked like a baby toadstool. People passing us were always like, "Oh she's so cute!" I was like, "I know...."

One time I was lying in bed with Joy for nap time, but she didn't seem tired. So we were going over what sounds different animals make. That was always so cute when we did that.

I remember playing hide and go seek with the girls in our house. Usually, they would hide in a closet. That was lots of fun. We often went to rivers and lakes and hiking trails all over Austin together. I had so much fun raising them for the 7 years that I did. But then it all went up in smoke, for many reasons.

Those memories are why I wanted to repeat all that with a new family, and now I am. Praise God for giving me another family. It is so wonderful to get to be a mother again.

Stolen Money

 Here is the craziest story that I have ever heard in my life. A family member that I know may have stolen 16k from her mom. Why did she? It makes no sense to me. She already has a free house from her mom. Her mom pays all her bills, as far as I know. The only thing she needs money for is food, but she has a boyfriend. Why isn't she just eating food at his place? She should have no need of 16k. I guess she just took it because she is greedy. She is the kind of person that always wants more. Maybe she is tired of waiting for her mom to die. It is like the story of the prodigal son in the Bible. He could not wait for his dad to die, so he asked for his share of the inheritance early. That is highly insulting to do that, because how do you know that your parent won't need that money for medical expenses? No one knows how long they will live.

Please pray with me that this mom will confront her daughter, even if she's scared to, and get her money back. She might really need that money back. Either way that is beyond messed up for a daughter to steal that much from her mom. Does she really not care about their friendship that much that she would steal that much? That is very mean.

I have never stolen anything from anyone, and I never would.

Ok I will say I had an 8k balance on a credit card a few years ago. They threatened to sue me or something, so I paid back half of it with a tax return, and they called it even. Technically I didn't pay it all back, so it was kind of like stealing from the credit card company. I guess they just figured any payment was better than nothing. Why did I max out an 8k credit card? My husband was too crazy to work. That was our only money for about 5 months. My mom paid our mortgage, but for anything else I used that. Looking back, I can't believe my ex didn't work for 5 months. Who does that when they have kids? It's no wonder why I was pretty angry at him in that time period.

Ah money...may God help us all to be more content with less so we will never steal from anyone ever. May I forgive myself for maxing out that credit card. It was crazy that I did that. But it's in the past. Hopefully I will never need a credit card ever again.

And hopefully this crazy daughter will start working instead of stealing money from her mom. Pray for her. Thanks all.

Toxic People

If you want a happy life, avoid toxic people.

Toxic people get bored easily because they don't have a hobby or a job that serves others. Therefore they start drama in any way they can. They love disaster and mayhem. They love destroying other people's lives. That is the most entertaining thing ever for them.

Misery loves company. They want others to feel as sad and lonely as they feel, so they break up relationships whenever they can.

Toxic people are boundary violaters. They don't care what you want. They only want what they want, when they want it.

They have been spoiled a ton. They spoil themselves and others have spoiled them. They are used to getting pretty much anything they want any time they want it. They do not respect anyone else. They don't really respect themselves either, because they know they cause others lots of pain. They seem to be in love with themselves, but really they hate themselves. They hate how they treat others, but it is almost impossible for them to change and be nice.

They lie and steal any chance they get. They only care about themselves.

If you are ever around toxic people, just ignore their crazy behavior. Don't let their madness make you go insane too. Focus on something else, like learning new health tips on the Jay Shetty show.

Time to Exercise

My Father's Day present to my man was to order roller blades. I am determined to get back in shape for him, and myself. :) The tricky thing about exercise is it makes you more hungry, but if you eat back all the calories you burn, you won't lose weight. I have been trying to not eat after 5pm. That only works some days. If I can pull off that rule and exercise, I'm sure I will get back in shape soon.

I hope we will skate around the biggest park in our city two days a week. That is my work out plan. I have never loved gyms very much, because I am a germaphobe. Can you imagine how many germs are at a gym? I can just smell them when I go into one.

So outdoor exercise will be great for our relationship! I roller skated today, and he rode his skateboard. I beat him lol. But roller blades are always faster than skateboards. It was super fun. At one point the sprinklers were on. It was a bit slippery, but I did not fall. Thank you God.

I tried the skate park there. I went down some ramps but ended up on my stomach in the grass. It was very sad. I didn't get hurt physically, but my pride was a bit hurt. It is tricky to be on roller blades.

I started learning to roller blade when I was only 6. My brother used to pull me around with his bike. I remember falling a lot and skinning my knees. I was too cool to wear knee pads. I was determined to learn how to roller blade super well.

I think I became interested in roller blading from the movie Free Willy. There is the movie scene where the kids are in a skate park, and it looked really cool to me. Today was my first time attempting to do a skate park. Usually I just stay on sidewalks. In California I went roller blading on the boardwalk next to the beach a lot. That was always a lot of fun. Here in Texas at least we have a super fun park to skate around. It was about 2 miles to skate around the entire park. I'll be in shape soon doing that twice a week. Woot!

What do you like to do for exercise? It is nice to do something every week. The more exercise I get, the better I feel. The endorphins are released and I feel on top of the world! Plus, it takes me back to my childhood when I played basketball a lot. I love that worn out feeling. It feels great!

May God inspire you to exercise in some way. It is good for everything, your mind, body and soul. It will make you much happier, even if it hurts a bit while you are exercising. No pain, no gain right? Get out there and have some fun!

May God bless you all.

Flashbacks

When I met my bf Zach I asked if his birth name was Zachariah. It was Zachary. Close enough! My birth name was Elizabeth. In the Bible those two have a son, and they name him John. I told him, "Maybe if we have a son we will name him John like Elizabeth and Zachariah did." He liked that idea. That was like the second day we met up. I guess I was hoping we would have a son from the very beginning.

But then I was thinking my baby would be a girl. I wanted to fully replace my two daughters. God asked me a few times though, "Do you want a boy so you have a different experience?" I said, "Ok that is fine."

It is better to have a son this time I think. It is nice that things are different. I feel more inclined to hug him. I don't know if it's because he is a boy or just that I am older and more loving now. It might also be that I am just happier now with my current man and our life. Our home I have made very happy with cute home decor. We have a beautiful backyard that I have worked hard on. Everything I could ever want is here. Except a bike. I still want to find a great bike.

I keep having PTSD though in regards to my baby. I keep being worried that things that happened to my first two girls will also happen to him. When Serenity, my first daughter, was about 2 she rolled off my bed. We were all playing and the girls were playing hide and go seek under the blanket. Serenity started rolling and rolled right off the bed onto the hard wood floor. I hope that didn't affect her brain forever. Now I am overly cautious with having my baby boy on an adult bed, as I should be.

Another time my second born, Joy, rolled off a changing table. Luckily it was onto carpeted floor. There was a bar on the side but she rolled right over the bar. Now I worry if my baby is ever on the changing table. Most kids don't do risky things like that but you never know.

I plan to never get a scooter or a bike for my baby boy. When Serenity was 5 she fell off her scooter pretty hard. We were on a bike trail and she went down a hill on her scooter. I thought she could handle it, but she wasn't an Olympic athlete like I literally saw her as. She lost balance at the bottom of the long hill and fell on her forehead. That was probably the incident that broke our whole family up. Maybe I was mad at my ex and he was mad at me for not telling her to walk down that hill.

It is hard to be a parent. One minute with them can change their entire life, and your entire life. She healed ok. I put ice on the bump on her head when we got home. But still, it was a very hard day for all of us.

Another day, months before that, Joy fell off her bike. She teetered over and fell at the end of the driveway, because driveways have those retarded mini hills on the sides. The handle bar fell on her finger and her fingernail cut her finger kind of badly. We took her to the ER for stitches. That was probably the scariest day of my life. It was just her finger but still, I freaked out.

So never again will I give a kid a scooter or a bike. I'm sure my boy could get hurt in other ways, but hopefully he won't. Maybe he will live a totally sheltered and perfect life. If he ever does get hurt, may

God help me to handle it with peace. But mostly I just hope he will never get hurt.

A Crazy Dream

I had a crazy dream last night about trying to go in and steal my two daughters. In my dream I was at my in law's house with my ex and my girls. Tons of other people were there too though. It turned into a movie like Mission Impossible. I was trying to take them away, but I got stopped and then people chased me for a long time trying to kill me. I suppose that is why I haven't tried to have shared custody. I would be tempted to just steal them away and who knows who would try hunting me after that. There is a movie like that kind of called Enough with Jennifer Lopez.

It gets messy when you decide to have kids with someone. If things don't work out with the partner, then what?

My mom took me away from my dad when I was 14. She wanted to live by her mom in CA again. I'm surprised she didn't take me away from him long before that. I remember driving away from his house with my mom and he was on his knees crying with my step-mom. There was nothing he could do. I didn't realize then that would be me someday. Maybe it was karma in a sense. I didn't care about leaving my dad and then my girls didn't care about leaving me. I'm sure they did a little, but I kept praying they wouldn't miss me too much, so maybe that prayer came true.

You can't hold onto anyone in life forever. I thought I could with my mom, but once your parent marries your step-parent you basically lose them. I haven't had my mom since she married my step-dad.

Hopefully my son and my current man will stay in my life forever. Pray for my man to not take too many pills. He is the kind of person that takes a pill for every kind of pain he has. I hope he doesn't give his body too much someday. Thank you for praying.

Spoiled Kids

 If there was a good reason for me giving up my two girls, it was that I knew I was making life too easy for them. They were spoiled, in the sense that I wanted to keep them babies forever. They drank out of bottles until age 3. They had food too, but I didn't know a clean way to let them have milk. That is odd I realize that. I couldn't find a good sippy cup and our house was new so I didn't want them spilling milk all over the new carpet. So I suppose I gave up my kids because I loved our house more than them. It was a beautiful house. Maybe that is why God gave me an average looking house now, so I won't overly love my house anymore.

I was very soft with my girls, too soft. I think most parents of girls are though. I had a horrible childhood and I wanted theirs to be comfortable and happy always. What I feared most was them having a bad childhood too. It seems to happen that what we fear the most, we bring about. Maybe that is because we think about it a lot. What you focus on is what will happen.

I had a great fear that my daughters would get sexually molested and one did. I had a great fear that they would be raised in a broken home and now they are.

Fear does not make us prevent bad things. Maybe it attracts bad things.

The hard times were also due to generational curses. The Bible says the sins of the father will affect the family for several generations. It is possible that my girls were cursed due to my dad's sin. He was a sex addict.

I think those curses have ended now. That only applies to the non saved people. So all y'all, make sure you are saved. I am now fully saved. It has been a recent development. I am confident that my son will not be affected by any of my family's generational curses. Praise God! I believe that my second family try will go well, and that it will last forever.

Choices

 This may sound odd but about 10 months ago God told me either I could start seeing my daughters every week, or I could be an artist. I chose to be an artist. That sounds messed up, but that was my decision.

What kind of artist? I was painting a ton at the time. Then I wrote about 10 books on great topics. Who knows what form of art I'll do next.

I've always wanted to be a famous singer. I think that is still possible. Sometimes I like writing songs.

Why did I have kids when I had so many dreams? I was willing to forget about my dreams for a season. I suppose every parent forgets their dreams for a long time, possibly forever. But having kids is worth it. What if you never could become famous? Then you are glad you didn't hang onto that dream forever.

I hope my daughters are doing well. I pray for them every day. I hope someday they will both meet happy and kind Christian men that they will live with and be willing to love forever.

If I ever see them again I would tell them, sorry I had to go live a separate life from your dad. He got to be too much for me to handle. His demonic possession was more than I could deal with. I hope your grandma kept you safe, even though you had to live with him. This world is crazy at times. Make a wise choice with the man you marry. I'm sorry that I didn't. And please don't become lesbian. □ There are great guys out there. Just listen to your gut feeling about him. You will find a great guy eventually. I love you both very much. I will always cherish the sweet memories of when I was raising you both.

A Time to Smile

 I have never had someone smile at me a lot. I have never had a guy that was totally smitten by me that he smiled a lot. I have never smiled a lot. That might be why. I have always been very serious, so everyone I came in contact with became serious around me.

Finally I get to see someone smile a lot. My little baby loves to smile at me and laugh. It might be because we watch Comedy sometimes. He hears people laughing so he wants to laugh. It is adorable.

I never heard my first two babies laugh. Maybe I just didn't believe they would and so they didn't. It was a very serious time back then. There wasn't much to smile or laugh about for any of us.

Now things are happy and fun and carefree. Praise God for the happy life and the happy baby I have now. If you are around a baby, make them laugh. They can do it.

Pain Leads to Maturity

"Consider it pure joy whenever you face trials of many kinds, because you know that the testing of your faith produces perseverance. Let perseverance finish its work so that you may be mature and complete, not lacking anything."

Am I more mature now after all my trails? Yes, a lot.

What have my trials been? Terrible migraines, loosing my kids and a few exes, loosing my house, conflict with most people I have known, a hard C Section, gall stones, a few near death experiences, a horrible dad....

Was it all good or bad? God said he works all things for the good for those who love him. Those trials were not good at all, but God can work it all for my good.

My ex died which was sad, but he was infertile. If he didn't die I never would have gotten to enjoy being a mother. Another ex left me, but that made it possible for me to inherit a free house.

God gives and he takes away. But still blessed be his name. He can do whatever he wants with our lives. We are here to serve him. If he needed to humble me through all those adversities, so be it.

Our character is more important than things we have or people we know. If we need to be molded by our creator more, he should be able to do anything he needs to with us.

Let God transform you through hard times. We learn the most in painful situations.

Money and Vaccines

I have wondered for a while now why on earth my mom would marry two child molesters in a row. I just had a thought. Essentially my dad cheated on my mom with me. I can't imagine how much that must have wrecked her self-esteem. Anytime someone gets cheated on, it makes you feel retarded. If it's a kid I'm sure the person feels even more retarded. It was probably from that need to have her insecurity go away that she decided to stick with my step-dad. She thought she couldn't do better. She knew he was accused of molesting his son by his ex-wife, but she chose to ignore it. He said it was a lie and she gullibly believed him. It was also the money he had that she wanted, and the love of money is the root of all evil.

Any time you hear about some pop star selling their soul to Satan you wonder why? Why would someone do that? It's the money. Satan, or some career executive, flashes a ton of cash at them if they will do this, this and that and they cave in. What is your price? What amount will make you do anything other people want you to do?

I was faced with a bribe lately to do something I didn't feel was ok. It felt like a bribe to sell my soul to Satan for money. There is no price I can put on what I believe in to be good. No amount of money would make me change my mind on what is good. What happened was my bf's grandma tried to bribe me to get my son vaccinated. She offered me $700 if I would allow him to get shots. In the moment I felt very much that it was like cases when people sell their soul to Satan for money. I had never been bribed before like that. I said no of course.

If you believe strongly about something, like I believe firmly that babies should not get vaccines, don't sell out for money. Don't give in just because that is what others want. Don't let people buy you out.

Whatever you might buy with that money does not compare with having the peace that you did the right thing.

Riches are temporary. Family is forever. Your faith is forever, or it should be. Stand your ground on things you believe in. It is worth the fight.

Good and Terrible Dads

 I have only seen one really outstanding dad in my life time. It was my first serious bf Roger. He willingly drove 3 hours in total every week just to see his two kids. He was an amazing dad.

My ex was and is a horrible dad. He doesn't care that our daughters never get to see me. That qualifies him as a terrible dad. When the family was still intact, almost all he did was watch porn in his room and neglect our kids and me. Or he stayed up really late playing a video game. That led to him missing a lot of sleep. This lack of sleep possibly was the source of him going insane.

My dad was terrible since he had a fetish for kids. Same with my step-dad. Both of them were hard workers but had serious sexual issues.

I wish dad's could try harder to be good dads, but it is rare to find a great one.

If God has blessed you with kids, be a good parent. It's not that hard.

My mom was lucky enough to have a Christian father. Was he a great father? It's hard to say. He was a good grandpa for me. For a while he basically was my dad, and I will always be grateful to him for filling that place of my father.

My current man is a good dad. He is willing to work long hours to be a great provider. He is very gentle with our son. Good job Zach!

May God help all the dads of the world to try harder. The world would be much better if dad's would try a lot more to be good fathers.

3 great movies y'all need to watch about being a good father...Mr. Mom, Daddy's Home and The Delivery Man. All of those are very well done movies.

Women Have Lost

 I wrote a book about Feminism called Feminism Sucks. Look it up on Amazon. It is listed under Lisa Bedrick books.

I was analyzing how most women have to decide between a career or raising kids. The issue in our modern world though is that women are doing both. So many women have abandoned the home and instead focus on making money. Then others don't respect them, and they don't respect themselves as much. It is like they are running away. They don't want to clean their house. They want to pay someone else to clean it. They don't want to raise their kids. They want a nanny or a daycare to raise their kids. No daycare worker will care about your kids as much as you do.

Women are leaving their natural duties to chase money. What do they have in the end? They feel less in touch with their kids. Kids are now running wild because too many women are chasing money instead of bonding with their kids.

Whatever you want to buy, is it really that important? Aren't your kids more important?

We wonder why kids are so messed up these days. It is because their mothers have run away from them. They are home but not really home. Or they are just never home.

Stay home women. Raise your kids yourself. No amount of money can replace the time with your kids. Before you know it, they will be gone. You will wish you would have focused on them more and not money.

Men, step it up and provide well for your families. If you want your wife to do a great job raising the kids, then you have to do a great job providing for them. You can do it. I believe in you.

Forgive Them

I think a lot of marriage conflict is due to anger that each has at the opposite sex. I used to make bracelets a lot. I am sure that is the main reason I have arthritis issues and that triggered the pre-clampsia that I had. I put on a bracelet one time, "Forgive Him." I felt like that was a word from the Lord. I have so many him's that I need to forgive. Almost every him I have known, I need to forgive.

My dad molested me. My brother did too. Another older guy did. All the guys who broke my heart I need to forgive. I still need to forgive my ex for letting his mind go insane and causing our family break up. My grandpa for speaking harshly at times. Guys that I worked with who were demeaning toward me.

I am sure every guy has a lot of hers that he needs to forgive. The start of most relationships is both people talking about their exes and how they were hurt by them. You help each other heal from all the previous pain. You assure each other that you will never hurt them like that other person did.

There is always so much pain to heal from.

May God help you all heal from your own pain from the opposite sex. Let those people go. Don't let them continue to hurt you by remembering what they did to you. Forgive and forget, when you are ready to.

Time or Money

Every woman wants both time and money from the man she is with. I used to think with my ex that if I didn't get his time, then I should get his money. You can't have a ton of both. You have to pick wanting more time or more money.

I used to want mainly just time with my current man more than money. Now since having a baby, money seems to be more important, but now I feel like I hardly ever see him. I heard in a sermon once that after having kids every woman forgets her man and focuses on her kids. Every man tends to forget his woman and focus just on working hard. Kids do divide couples. This is why it can be harder to spend a lot of time as a couple before having kids. If you want kids, just have them, so you don't get too used to spending time with your mate. Things are very different after having kids. I remember before I got pregnant God told me, "He doesn't realize having a kid will mean he has to say goodbye to you." I didn't get what God meant. Working more hours is probably what he meant. Ironically my son's name James means "supplanter." To supplant means to replace something. I used to hang out with my man all day when he worked less hours. Now I hang out with baby James all day.

Money has to be made though. Formula isn't cheap. Diapers get expensive. Although I found a good brand that isn't too pricey. Get Parent's Choice diapers if you have a baby. They are good enough quality and super cheap.

I got used to having a lot of alone time with my man before having a baby too. He is on an anti-depressant which makes him think and feel like he needs 12 hours of sleep every night. So every morning for over a year now I have had lots of alone time, hence all my writing. I can only hope the books I wrote will help people. Hopefully the effort was well worth it. May God multiply my efforts.

I can't sleep 12 hours. I am always up around 6 or 7am no matter what. It's too bad there isn't a home job I could do in the morning. I suppose this writing is my work. It is my volunteer work that God willing helps all you who read it.

If you are frustrated over wanting both time and money from your mate, I understand. Try to figure out what you want more. If you want more time, then spends less money so they can work less.

Boys Have More Fun

 Have you ever known a really fun woman? Probably not. That is because women just Want to have fun, but only boys Know how to have fun. Us women are so serious. Little girls are serious. If we are having fun, it is by trying to impress other people. That is what is fun for us. But it isn't really fun because we are hoping for a good job. Most of the time we don't get that, so it isn't fun anymore. So sad....

Men usually don't care about impressing others. They just have fun. They know how to relax. Women have a hard time relaxing. Even after I had C Section surgery, I had a hard time relaxing. There is always something to do. The grass needs to be watered. The floors need to be cleaned. The laundry needs to get done. We can never just be totally chilled out.

I could have told them that in the hospital. They asked often why my blood pressure was so high. It is because I always think of things that need to get done. There is always something to do. Men only do a lot of things when women tell them to.

My son is 2.5 months old now, and he smiles a ton. He is working on his laugh too. My two daughters almost never smiled or laughed as babies. It might be that I was overly serious back then though. When my oldest was a baby, I was always busy trying to publish books. I was organizing these blogs into books and publishing as many as I could. Other than that, I was just concerned with caring for her, but I didn't have fun with her. I didn't enjoy being a mom to her per say.

When my second girl was a baby, we had a crazy bug issue. I was always worried about cleaning and trying to get rid of them. They were white fuzzball bugs that invaded any home we had and my car. It took me years to get rid of them. So I was always stressed out over that. I suppose the level of joy a mom has will be the level of joy her baby has.

I think a woman's mood when she is pregnant also matters. I have heard it does anyways. I was pretty happy in this last pregnancy. My heartburn was annoying, but I kept thinking of fun book topics and writing everything about every hot topic I could think of. That was tons of fun.

In my first two pregnancies I wasn't very happy. I found out my ex was talking to other girls online. In both pregnancies I was far away from my mom, which was sad. I didn't call people very much just to chat. This last pregnancy I called friends a lot. When my son was born, he was looking at me like, "I heard you talking a lot when I was on the inside of you, and now I can see you! Yay...."

He is so cute. We have a great friendship already. I hope my boy and I will be best friends forever. And I hope he will always have tons of fun.

Pros and Cons of Raising my Baby

Here is something that is crazy. We are spending $14 a day on formula. But of course, our little adorable baby is worth every cent.

I am on my own on the night shift. I slightly resent that, so I buy myself happy things sometimes to say good job to myself for doing that. You always see in movies that both the mom and dad are sleep deprived due to caring for the baby. Nope, it's just me. I didn't expect my bf to wake up for the baby though because my ex never did for my daughters. I don't know how common it is for dads to be willing to miss sleep for their baby. Maybe half of dads are willing to. It depends on the job they have I would think. If their job requires a lot of energy from them, they probably won't wake up to help the mom at night.

My grandmother in law seems to be addicted to having time with the baby. She is 83 though, so eventually I will have to tell her she is too old to hold him. I don't have the guts to tell her that yet. Please pray for me on that. Thanks all.

My mother in law watches the boy 3 days a week at her house. That is great, and I appreciate her doing that very much. It gives me and my bf time to catch our breath and just relax together again. So nice.

Baby James is not spitting up as much now. Thank you God for that.

I used to go on walks with him in the stroller. I should try doing that again. It has been 108 every day here lately, so walks seem a bit undoable. I hope the weather cools off a bit soon.

Every day we watch music videos and comedy from Drybar together. I nap on the couch if he is napping. He likes to actually watch the TV already so that is fun. Maybe someday he will become a comedian or a country singer. How cool would that be.

Overall it has been fun raising my boy so far. I have good help and a fair amount of money to work with. It is a good life that I have set up for myself here.

Formula vs. Breastfeeding

I have regretted a few times that I did not try breastfeeding my baby more. He was a primi though, so he seemed too weak to breastfeed at first. Also when you are in the hospital, they feed the babies formula from day one. I think how things used to be was that the baby had to get so hungry that they felt they had to figure out how to breastfeed. If the baby isn't really hungry, they aren't very motivated to breast feed. Hospitals should probably consider that. It is good to feed the baby something obviously, but when formula takes the place of the mom from the beginning, it is hard to train the baby to breastfeed.

I tried getting two different breast pumps. It was a very slow process to pump. I had in laws over all day, every day so that made it hard to get time to pump. It wasn't their fault though. That was mandated by CPS. The cause of that mainly was jealousy from a night nurse there. She started drama for me by complaining to CPS about me. I think it was mainly because I was white. Perhaps she hates white people.

About pumping, I should have shut myself in a room more often to get that done but I didn't. I also have neck issues from accidents as a kid, and pumping hurt my neck a lot.

I wish breast feeding would have worked out though because it was free milk. Formula is crazy expensive, unless you get the powdered kind, but then the baby might not get all that full. I use the pre-mixed kind which might be made with soy milk.

I hope the formula is totally safe for the baby. There are strange things in some baby products, possibly due to the elite's desire to depopulate. I hope there is nothing dangerous in the formula I am giving to my son.

If you use formula for your baby, don't worry. It is hard to do everything perfectly as a mom. Let yourself off the hook of that expectation. Forgive yourself. Obviously breastfeeding is ideal, but not everyone can pull it off. May God give you peace about whatever you decide to feed your baby.

God bless and good luck fellow moms.

The Best Way to Feed a Baby

It is tricky to know when to feed a baby and how much. Generally, it is best to wait for them to cry for a feeding time. If they aren't really hungry, then there is no point in making a bottle. It is important though that babies have a small bottle at least once every 2 hours. Most of us adults like to eat at least a snack every 2 hours. Babies are the same way. Small feedings often are ideal for them, and us.

This blog will mostly be about formula feeding. I think with breastfeeding it takes about 90% of the baby's day. Good job to you ladies that breastfeed, but that is one reason I have never been all that inclined to breastfeed. It takes a lot longer to get the baby full.

With formula feeding, there is the stress of finding a great bottle. I like the Dr. Brown bottles. It takes a bit of time for the baby to get used to different bottles. It is ideal to stick with the same kind forever. If you feed the baby too much, they might throw up, or they will have lots of spit up. It is better to do small feedings but more frequently. Then they spit up less, which is so nice.

When my baby was born, he was a primi so he was very skinny. Of course that made me sad, and my main goal then was to make him fat. Now he has a double chin. I am very happy about that. A lot of work went into his double chin.

It is ideal to stick with the same formula forever also. The more you change formula brands, the more it can mess up the baby's digestion of the formula.

Try getting your baby to hold his bottle as soon as possible. It is very hard to do feedings in the middle of the night. If you can just hand your baby a bottle, that will help you get a lot more sleep. Keep the amount of formula low for middle of the night feedings. They usually just want a snack but not a full meal during the night time.

May God bless your baby, and may he or she gain weight appropriately.

Kid Sports

 I will probably have my son try all the same sports that I did, in the order that I did them. I had a lot of fun growing up playing tons of sports.

My first sport, or form of good exercise, was bike riding. I might skip that one for him though. Bikes caused me and my daughter serious injuries. Bikes can be incredibly dangerous. Maybe that is why currently, my in laws discouraged me from bike riding.

When I was 6, I was on a swim team. That was very therapeutic for me. I had a hard childhood, but I think that kept me happy. In 4th grade I started basketball, volleyball and soccer. I just did soccer for a year, but it was still fun. I played volleyball for 3 years. I was pretty good.

Basketball I kept playing for the next 12 years. I played on teams in school and then intramural in college. I played at parks a lot, usually with all guys. That was lots of fun. They were always enamored that a female could really play well. That was always a fun ego boost for me.

I played softball for one summer after 7th grade. My team was all my friends from school so that was super cool.

I never tried playing tennis on a team, but I played for fun a lot in my 20's.

The only sports I have never played are water polo and normal golf. I have done mini golf many times, as most of us have.

One of my dreams is to open an indoor air conditioned mini golf course. Maybe someday I will. That is great family boding time.

I suppose a great first sport for boys is T ball. That would be cute to see my son play that. I hope he enjoys sports just as much as I always did. May God bless him with great athletic talent so the sports will be a lot more fun for him. And may God bless your kids and grandkids with great athletic skill also.

Medical Bills

I have no intention of paying my medical bill from my C Section. I feel slightly bad about that, but it is my decision. I gave that hospital 1k, which was money a family member generously gave me, in advance for my bill. I feel like that is what it should cost for a C Section, and that is what I paid them. They kept me for 6 days against my will. When you have a C Section, you can't just leave anytime. They have to release you.

Granted I had high blood pressure, but I could have gone home sooner. Doctors get way too paranoid about blood pressure. They were just being greedy maybe. Perhaps someone thought, "Ha the longer we keep her, the higher her medical bill will be, and we will all get bonuses."

 I would have wanted to go home right after my C Section. My mother in law could have been my free nurse. And she wouldn't have been drawing my blood every day and waking me up a lot. I appreciate all they did, but it wasn't necessary. Why should any of us pay for medical care that we don't want or need? That is probably why most people don't pay their medical bills. Also, if they weren't so high, we would pay them. I know they are so high because very few people pay them. Essentially when you pay a medical bill, you are paying for 10 other people too who didn't pay theirs.

Other countries are very wise with this. They raise taxes and that covers any medical expense. That is what we should do too. I think taxes are currently about 30% of someone's income. That should cover medical expenses. If it doesn't, then that is just ridiculous.

Someday I might pay all the medical bills I still owe. I might get a giant inheritance soon and then I probably will in order to raise my credit score. For now, I don't care much about my credit score. I have a paid off car, and I plan to live in my free house the rest of my life. Good credit is not really needed for anything else.

The nurses kept wondering why my blood pressure was high. I said one time, "Maybe if you guys would let me nap, it would go down." But they come in your room every 20 minutes for a different reason. It was fun to be more social with 30 different people though. That part was fun. The chef lady calls to get your order for every meal. I wish every day of my life was like that. I couldn't taste the food very well though due to the blood pressure meds they had me on. That was sad.

It was nice having the nursery at night. I did feel God told me to be willing to stay for 6 days, mainly to spread some light there, but also to recover fully before doing the night baby shift on my own. Sometimes I would play worship music in my hospital room. I realized that might cause some spiritual attack, which it did.

My bf stayed the night with me there every night, which was nice. One night I attempted to cuddle with him in the almost twin sized hospital bed. That was interesting.

It was mostly a good experience, but I still don't feel inclined to pay the bill for it. I paid 1k. That is how much it should have been. If you have medical bills and you need good credit, pay them. Even if you pay just $20 a week, they can't send it to collections. May God bless you with wisdom about what to do about your medical bills. God bless.

Money

 Rich people never stop working. If you want to acquire great wealth, work like a dog every single day doing something. You never know when your hard work will really pay off.

Rich people invest in houses. If you ever have extra money, buy a house. Buy 10 houses. The game of monopoly taught us all that.

Rich people don't care about money as much you might think they do. The more you care about money, the harder it will be to get. Think of what you want to do with your money rather than the money itself. Then you will accomplish that goal.

What would Jesus do? Was he rich? No, not necessarily, but he never went hungry, except when he was fasting on purpose. Jesus always had his needs met. Why? Because he was always doing something. "A teacher is worthy of his wages." He taught. He healed. He was always busy. There wasn't a lazy day for Jesus. He never just slept all day. He never just did nothing for a long time. He was either praying or helping others in some way.

If we all work like Jesus did, we will always have our needs met too. Never get lazy. Always try to help others in some way and then all your needs will get met too. Believe it and receive it.

Getting rich is not everything. The ultimate goal of life should be helping others. "Seek first the kingdom of God and all these earthly things will be added to you as well."

Keep working hard. Your hard effort will reward you eventually.

Dealing with a Mate with Autism

I wasn't sure if I should write about this, but there might be a lot of you out there who are dealing with an autistic mate or child. My bf is somewhat autistic. How do I know? He repeats himself a lot. Like he doesn't remember what he told me already. It is possible he just shrank his brain too much from smoking pot most of his life. He doesn't smoke it now. I think that is what people with disabled brains do to feel better though, or to unwind from the stress of being autistic.

How did he become autistic? His vaccines may have caused it a little. It may run in his family.

If you are wondering if your child or mate is autistic, look at their eyes. If their eyes seem kind of droopy, that is a sign of autism.

It is good to recognize that so you will be nicer to your autistic child, or your mate. Once you realize they really can't change the way they act, and they have little control over it, you will have more patience with them. Understanding helps to make us all more kind to others.

My brother also was always slightly autistic. For him I think it was his vaccines, but also the Ritalin that my parents put him on for several years. From age 9 till about 20 he was on a lot of Ritalin. One time he said to me, "Why can't you slow down?" I said to him, "Why can't you speed up?" And that was how things always were with us. I didn't get why he was slow, and it annoyed him that I was faster than him. That may have happened to prepare me for having a slightly autistic mate.

Despite all that, I love my man very much. It is possible that I love him even more because he is autistic. It makes him cuter, because he is more simple. He doesn't stress out about things as easily, like all us smart people do. He never worries about the future. He is always just very simplistic and low key. He is not complex at all, which is nice after all the complex and highly emotional guys I have been with. I never worry what he is thinking about, because it is always something simple.

What does he do for work? He is probably only able to do the job that he does, which is doing to go orders at a restaurant. I am ok with him not making tons of money, because he inherited a free house. The only thing he has to make money for is our food, so that is very good.

I think why God allows some people to be autistic is that it reminds the rest of us to just chill out, to not take life so seriously, to not worry about every little thing. It reminds us to focus on love and nothing else. Autistic people are very often some of the most loving and kind people, depending on the degree of autism they have. Nothing gets in the way of them loving you. They don't have thoughts against you, usually. They don't desire to argue with you or to always be the one who is right. They just are, and that is very cute and relaxing to be around.

If your mate or child are autistic, don't worry. They can still have a
fun and great life, and you can too. Just learn to appreciate the
different way their brain works, and then you will be victorious in
bonding with them well. Be kind to them, because they deserve a lot
of kindness. They mean you no harm. They are just different than the
rest of us, but in many ways, they are sweeter and cuter.

May God give you wisdom as you try to understand their different
way of thinking. You can do it. I believe in you.

Autism in My Family

I have always been concerned about this issue in our society. I
interacted with an autistic child at my church about 15 years ago. I
could not reason with him. It was like he didn't even speak english.
His mom was exhausted from having to deal with him.

I used to say I would not have a child after age 35 because the risk of
Autism increases. I just had my baby boy at age 38. I am quite sure
my baby boy does not have Autism though. He smiles and is
interactive with anyone talking to him. He looks smart. He makes eye
contact with me a lot. I can tell he is a totally healthy baby.

I was a bit extra worried though because I think my bf is Autistic. I
think it runs in his family blood line. It is possible that his mom is
Autistic and her mom may have been also.

I was reading the symptoms last night. Autistic people have
downward slanting eyes, so they look tired all the time. Another sign
is when someone is like a robot. They cannot connect emotionally
with others. They have almost no expressions. They never smile or
laugh. They cannot cry or really feel very much at all. Their voice is

monotone. They look very awkward in social interactions. My bf has all those symtoms.

It made me wonder if my step-dad is Autistic because he has all those symptoms too. It is possible he is slighly Autistic, because he has always been very awkward socially. I wonder if he got it from his mom.

Usually children get it from their mother. My ex mother in law I think was Autistic, but somehow neither of her kids turned out to be. At least it wasn't obvious if they were.

My brother was Autistic. Although with him, you can't see it in his eyes. He just had brain malfunctions. He was awkward socially. Usually he had no friends growing up, but he didn't seem to care. He got teased a lot. He had bad grades. He was not coordinated in sports.

My dad was labeled ADHD. He was hyper for sure, but that could have been due to the medications he was on. He was on Ritalin for a while just like my brother. They told me it speeds up their brain waves. I remember thinking, why would he need a drug to speed him up when he already is sped up?

I realized last night that almost everyone seems to be either ADHD or Autistic. Either they are very energetic, or they seem to have no energy. Of course that could just be the extroverts and the introverts. Extroverts seem always full of energy. They could pretty much all be labeled as ADHD. Introverts always seem tired, and they prefer to be alone. They feel awkward in social situations. They could almost all be labeled as Autistic.

I suppose no one knows how to treat any of these brain illnesses fully. I think about half of America has something wrong with their brain. Why? Healthcare. Doctors have messed up so many people with their drugs and procedures. It is very hard to keep your brain normal in our modern world. I read that even air pollution can cause Autism. That could affect all of us.

Keep your head on straight. Keep eating healthy so any toxins in the environment won't mess with your brain. Stay away from any and all drugs. Then your brain will always run well and you will never seem to have a brain disability.

Autism Can be Fixed

The more socialization a person who is Autistic has, the less their Autism will affect them. An Autistic person is more inclined to isolate because they know they are different, but that is the worst thing for them to do. The only way to get better at interacting with others is to interact more with others.

Autistic people are more prone to anxiety or depression. I never thought I would recommend medication, but it can help those who are Autistic. They are more prone to temper tantrums. If they are on a medication, it helps to calm them down a lot.

I worked with a guy who was Autistic for about 2 years. He had some pretty big temper tantrums. I couldn't tell what was wrong with him. I am finally realizing that it was Autism. He never smiled or laughed. He didn't seem to have empathy with anyone, which made him a good manager actually, because he forced us all to work harder. Yes I had an Autistic manager at a pizza store. That was quite difficult at times.

"Those who need love the most, deserve it the least." Autistic people often do not get much love, because they do not know how to show love. It is very hard for them to express the love that they feel. They might feel just as much love as anyone does, but they don't know how to express it. To be in a relationship with an Autistic person, you have to see past their actions. You have to be able to read their heart. It is a kind of deep intuition to be able to do this. They come off as not caring about anyone, but that is not the truth about them. The more you show them how to show love, the better they will understand how to show love.

I remember being disappointed that my daughters never said, "I love you Mom." But to be fair I never said to them, "I love you Joy (or Serenity)." I don't know why I didn't say that. I suppose because my mom didn't say that very much to me. And her mom was raised in an orphanage. So the lack of affirmation and affection carried down the family line. When you are not shown how to love, it is hard for you to show love later on. If you want your child to hug you, hug them a ton first. If you want them to say "I love you," say "I love you" to them first a lot.

It is the same with Autistic people. In many ways, they are still a child on the inside. They take longer to learn things and to mature. Some poeple it seems like are born mature. They learn fast, and they know how to do everything very quickly. I was always a quick learner. Others take years to learn things. Their brain is defective. They cannot help it. They would love to learn faster, but they can't.

I know a woman who was probably born Autistic. Her eyes are slanted down, so she must have inherited it from a family member. You can't tell hardly at all that she is Autistic. She seems to have outgrown it. She has had enough social interactions by now that it almost doesn't affect her at all. Or she has just learned well how to pretend to be normal. She might not feel normal, but she comes off as very normal.

It just takes Autistic people longer to mature. I always heard girls mature 2 years faster than boys. Normal people mature about 10 years faster than Autistic people.

It is hard for Autistic people to talk. The more chances they get to talk, the better they will get at talking. The main reason I can talk for hours, or write for hours, is due to all the counseling I have gone through in my life. I have seen about 8 different counselors about being sexually molested as a child. That also can take away your desire to communicate. You can then also stay frozen as a child. I had to work at maturing at a normal pace I suppose. The counseling helped me to mature faster and understand myself more and become more confident. Anyone who struggles with self-esteem should see a counselor. It is great to pay someone to listen to you talk for a long time. It makes you realize you can have some interesting things to say. It helps you learn to trust others again as your counselor reacts positively and compassionately to things you say.

I remember one time giving my testimony in India on a missions trip. I shared about my dad sexually molesting me and my youth pastor had the most compassionate look on her face. It almost made me cry. It was nice to see someone who really cared about that. I was so used to people not caring that much, or at least no one showed me they cared all that much. My mom was callous to the situation. My brother never said anything to me about it. My grandmothers never spoke to me about it. It was like no one really cared that it happened. And then I saw her look, and I saw compassion about it for the first time in my life. I think that helped me decide to trust people again. She helped for a few years to reverse the damage that my dad did to me. She loved me out of my mistrust of people. She showed me that some people can be really good.

The same can be done for Autistic people. Maybe a lot of people have hurt them since they seem different. All it takes is one or two people to love them really well and they can get better and feel better. They can desire to interact with others more. They will want to be more social. They will learn to trust others again. If you treat them like you treat eveyone else, eventually they will start to be just like everyone else.

Kids Cause a Goodbye

Before I got pregnant I felt like God said to me, "He doesn't realize this will make him have to say goodbye to you." That was in reference to me getting pregnant and having Zach's baby. Why did God say that? Not that I would leave physically, but we barely see each other now.

Before I had our baby I would water the yard in the mornings, take a bath, and then come and cuddle with him. We pretty much never cuddle anymore. I always only cuddled with him in the mornings because he didn't snore then, for whatever reason. At night my man snores as loud as an airplane.

Now he has to work tons. He works 14 hour days 3 days a week, 7 hour days 3 days a week and only gets one day off. On that one day he is so tired all he wants to do is drink and sleep all day.

So children have a way of making couples say goodbye to each other, even though they are still technically together. This is why a lot of couples wait to have kids or never have kids. They know they will barely see each other afterwards. But that is life.

When I was younger I never wanted to have kids actually. One of my exes convinced me by saying, "Well who will take care of you when you are old?" I was like, "Ok, that is a good reason to have kids."

To all you fellow parents, I know how you feel if you miss your mate. Someday you will get to hang out with them again, when the kids are grown. Or when they are teens, and they want to have their own life apart from you. Hang in there and stay strong.

How Many Kids?

We are wondering now if we should have more kids, but what would be the reason to?

 I think one reason most parents have multiple kids is because they worry one of their kids will die or get paralyzed. The problem is though, the more kids you have, the greater risk of bad things happening to each of them.

They can hurt each other. You can't focus on each one individually for very long. One kid might dare another kid to do something stupid and dangerous. Or one just wants to prove he is just as cool as his brother so he does risky things. They compete for their parents favor, so they try to one up each other often.

I like the verse, "As iron sharpens iron so one man sharpens another." That verse is about siblings, I would say. They may make you sharper, but it hurts.

With multiple kids you get jealousy, competition, pushing each other down due to jealousy. The more kids, the more fighting over toys or food. Favoritism always happens when there is more than one. One kid feels special and the rest feel jealous and hate the special one. What did Joseph's brothers do? They tried to kill him.

So in light of all that, parents who only have one kid are the smartest. As long as that one kid stays alive and healthy, it is the best possible life a parent can have.

Goals

 When my son is around 16 and he has a girlfriend and has less time for me, I would love to get a Masters in counseling. Then maybe I could start my own counseling private practice for children. I have always wanted to counsel children of any age about abuse they endured. I know if I can say to them "I have been there" it would mean a lot to them. My dad attempted to rape me when I was 6.

My other big goal is to start a custom children's clothing store. I would use fabric paint and put encouraging phrases on kids' shirts, maybe Bible verses.

I also want to sail around the world on a cruise with my man and my son.

Maybe someday I can get full custody of my first two daughters again. I just need to have more money. Hey, go buy some of my other books.

My Testimony

I was raised in a very religious family. I say religious because my mom was Christian but my dad was just religious. They were involved in a church called "the Local Church" for a long time, which was very legalistic. The people may have looked good on the outside and said all the right stuff, but it was mostly goodness out of competition or fear I think.

My dad molested me for awhile in my childhood. I could never wrap my mind around how he could be Christian and do that, but he wasn't Christian, he was just religious. I have had a lot of anger at my mom throughout my lifetime about all that, mainly just at the fact that she married my dad. I felt she should have taken more time to really judge his character before marrying him, since obviously he turned out to be a bit crazy. He was analyzed by psychiatrists who said he was "highly intelligent but with a skewed sense of reality." That skewed sense was that he thought it was his job to teach me everything about life, including sexuality. Very skewed indeed.

He went to jail when I was 6 because I told my mom about something he did. She did not know the whole time what was happening. He was only in jail for a short time and our family reunited after he got out, which I also had anger at my mom about as an adult. If it were me, I would have never spoken to him again.

But then when I was 9 my parents divorced, praise God. Although that divorce was a bit hard on me. I started getting into a lot of trouble, shoplifting and drinking and smoking from about 12 to 14. Mainly it was because I felt that I was bad due to what happened to me so I thought I might as well act bad.

When I was 14 my mom and I moved to California from Nebraska to be by her parents. Praise God for that because from then on my grandma was a very strong and very positive influence in my life. She helped me see that I needed to do better and that God had a great plan for my life, despite what happened to me. I felt like she really believed in me, that I could do anything and be anything. So I did. I went on a mission's trip at 14 to India. I joined all the leadership teams at my church. I was in tons of AP classes in high school and a debate club and choir and basketball. I did everything I could do. I love a quote I heard once, "The most reprobate sinners become the most devout saints." I think it's because the energy you put into being bad you then put into doing good and helping others.

Then I went to Biola for college, a private Christian school. I kind of had the wind taken out of my sails there. I think I felt less than the other kids who all seemed to come from perfect families. I felt kind of like the black sheep there all four years. I also had lots of anxiety about what people thought of me and my grades. But I did learn a ton about the Bible and God there and I praise God for that.

After college I mostly worked at jobs helping kids. I felt like my calling in life was to help other kids have a really happy childhood since I didn't. I have heard "Your greatest ministry comes from your greatest pain." My greatest pain was that most of my young life was not happy at all, so I wanted to create happiness for as many kids as I could. I ran games at summer camps, tried teaching and did lots of tutoring. I tried to encourage as many kids as I could, like my grandma always had encouraged me.

At 25 I met a wonderful Christian guy. We got engaged, but when I was 27 he died due to drinking while on to many prescriptions. That started a war inside me kind of against prescription drugs and doctors. That time of grieving over his death was a very, very hard time for me. I never questioned my faith though. I only pressed harder into God in that time and started writing in my new blog a ton. His death made me realize even more how little time we all have, and that I could die any day. I felt all the more that I needed to start doing as much as I could to help others and change the world, as much as I could.

When I was 28 I met my ex-husband online. We had two little girls who were total angels. We divorced 3 years ago due to his mental health problems. He may have just been scientifically Schitzophrenic, or demons were pestering him in his mind. Whatever it was, we could not stay together. I did not feel safe living with him anymore, due to his involvement in Charismania. I felt that type of church was full of witchcraft and as a result, he seemed to become possessed.

About 9 years ago I started making something I call "Jesus Packets" that have bracelets, candy and a Bible tract. I think my motivation for those is that if I can't save my dad, maybe I can help to save many others. I think I have made about 8,000 of those so far. Hopefully those are making a difference. My goal in life has always been to push away the darkness as much as I can and shine as much light in this world as I can in any way I can, through music or making craft things or my blog writing. Hopefully God has taken every effort I have made and multiplied it's effects like Jesus did with the bread and the fish.

About 16 months ago I met my current sweetie. We both went to Christian school for a while growing up. We feel like a good match and God willing, we will stay together forever.

If you have never prayed to receive the free gift of Jesus' salvation, say this prayer, "God thank you for sending Jesus to die for me. Holy Spirit please come into my heart and transform me into the person God wants me to be."

Here is a good tip for you all. Something great to do in your free time is to start a Bible study habit. Search any topic on the website OpenBible.com. You can read every Bible verse that exists on any topic you may want to learn more about. May God bless you and your family!

About the Author:

Lisa Bedrick was born and raised in Orange County, CA. She currently lives in West Texas. She was saved at age 14 and went to a private Christian college. She has a B.A. in English. God is number one in her life. She met her man, Zach through online dating. He is a great Christian guy. They just had a wonderful baby boy that they named James.

Thank you for reading my book. God loves you!

www.ingramcontent.com/pod-product-compliance
Lightning Source LLC
Chambersburg PA
CBHW050051260726
48658CB00005B/1886